50 Ways to Abuse Your Voice

50 Ways to Abuse Your Voice

A Singer's Guide to a Short Career

Robert T. Sataloff, M.D., D.M.A, F.A.C.S.

Mary J. Hawkshaw, R.N., B.S.N., CORLN

Jaime Eaglin Moore, M.D.

Amy L. Rutt, D.O.

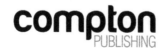
compton
PUBLISHING

Compton Publishing

This edition first published 2014 © 2014 by Compton Publishing Ltd.

Registered office: Compton Publishing Ltd, 30 St. Giles', Oxford, OX1 3LE, UK

Registered company number: 07831037

Editorial offices: 3 Wrafton Road, Braunton, EX33 2BT, UK

Web: www.comptonpublishing.co.uk

ISBN 978-1-909082-11-3

A catalogue record for this book is available from the British Library.

Cover illustration: Cover design: David Siddall, http://www.davidsiddall.com

Set in Adobe Caslon Pro 11pt by Regent Typesetting

1   2014

Contents

Preface

In 1985, the author (RTS) published an article called "Ten Good Ways to Abuse Your Voice: A Singers Guide to a Short Career, Part I" in the NATS Journal. The readers enjoyed the article, and it was followed in 1986 by "Ten More Good Ways to Abuse Your Voice: A Singers Guide to a Short Career, Part II." Singers have continued to send in comments expressing appreciation for these old articles which are now somewhat outdated. So, when Noel McPherson, owner of Compton Publishing, requested a book based on the concept of those articles, the idea seemed timely. The original articles have been updated and converted into new chapters. Thirty additional chapters have been added, some of which are completely new, and some of which were modified from prior writings. The authors are grateful to the publishers of our previous works for permission to republish and modify materials for inclusion in this book. We acknowledge the following sources:

Sataloff, R.T. *Professional Voice: The Science and Art of Clinical Care.* New York, NY: Raven Press; 1991.

Sataloff, R.T. *Professional Voice: The Science and Art of Clinical Care,* Second Edition. San Diego, CA: Singular Publishing Group, Inc.; 1997.

Sataloff, R.T. *Professional Voice: The Science and Art of Clinical Care,* Third Edition. San Diego, CA: Plural Publishing, Inc.; 2005.

Sataloff, R.T., Brandfonbrener, A. and Lederman, R. (Eds.). *Performing Arts Medicine*, Third Edition. Narberth, PA: Science and Medicine; 2010.

Smith, B. and Sataloff, R.T. *Choral Pedagogy*, Third Edition. San Diego, CA: Plural Publishing, Inc.; 2013

Journal of Singing, National Association of Teachers Singing (NATS).

This book is intended to provide straightforward, accessible information to singers, highlighting common errors of omission and commission, and to provide guidance on medical issues that affect the quality and duration of a career in singing. Unlike most of our medical writings, the chapters are short, and they are not heavily referenced or illustrated. Interested readers can find additional information and reference source materials in our other books (listed among the suggested readings at the end of this book) and in other sources. We hope that our readers find this work enjoyable and useful, and that the knowledge acquired through these pages helps enhance and extend their singing careers.

Robert Thayer Sataloff
Mary Hawkshaw
Jaime Eaglin Moore
Amy Rutt

To the thousands of singers for whom we have cared over the years. We have learned as much from them as they have from us.

To our families.

Acknowledgements

The authors are indebted to Christina Chenes and Deborah Keeler for their assistance in preparation of this book.

Don't warm up before you use your voice

Most trained singers will laugh at this admonition and say, "Of course I would never sing without warming up." However, the statement does not say "warm up before *singing*"; it says, "warm up before you use your voice." While very few trained singers would go out on stage to perform without having "warmed up," it is amazing how many singers will go through an entire day of heavy voice use in classrooms, teaching and other business situations without some vocal exercise (warm ups). Unfortunately, most singers "practice" in the afternoon and evening. Yet, if this follows a day of lecturing, teaching music classes, singing in choral rehearsals, etc., the practice comes too late. It is like warming up for the first time after running a marathon. Much can be gained by vocal exercises first thing in the morning. Even if a singer sings scales for only five to ten minutes to warm up, stretch and place the voice before beginning a day of speaking, the difference in vocal awareness, voice conservation, and control of the speaking voice may be substantial. We have personally cared for people prepared to retire from teaching or conducting because of hoarseness and vocal fatigue who have found morning vocal warm ups sufficient to restore them to good vocal performance.

2

Don't exercise

Singing is an athletic activity. Vocal exercise is as essential to the vocalist as exercise and conditioning of other muscle systems are to an athlete. Proper vocal practice incorporates scales and specific exercises designed to maintain and develop the vocal apparatus. Simply acting or singing songs and giving performances without routine, studious concentration on vocal technique usually is not adequate for the vocal performer. It requires excellent respiratory conditioning, endurance and good general health. This is true even of recital singing, let alone opera productions in which singing is combined often with running, dancing, fencing and other taxing activities. It is also true for pop and rock singing on which intense performance may be required for 6 sets 6 nights a week, and for "Broadway" or "West End" singing which often involves 8 shows a week. Obesity, poor general conditioning, avoidance of some form of aerobic exercise regularly, and failure to maintain good abdominal and thoracic muscle strength will undermine the power source of the voice and predispose the singer to vocal difficulties.

3

Don't study singing

There are many reasons why singers choose to not study singing or to stop taking singing lessons. In general, none of them are valid. Probably the most common reason for singers to refuse voice lessons is given by "pop" singers. They are often afraid that singing lessons will make them sound "operatic" and will interfere with their style. In the hands of a good teacher, this is not true. The same basic techniques of vocal production and voice preservation required of classical singers work for popular singers and may be used regardless of style. In fact, popular singers often need technical expertise at least as much as classical singers. Unfortunately, part of the blame for the "bad image" of voice teachers within the popular music community falls on the heads of our best voice teachers. Too often, our elite teachers refuse to teach singers interested in popular music careers, restricting their studios to "serious" singers. This forces popular singers to study with less knowledgeable teachers, stylists who call themselves teachers, or worse. Popular singers, whose livelihoods depend upon their voices and music (and whose economic potential may be very substantial), have received less than their fair share of attention; and it is past time for expert singing teachers to reassess their willingness to teach them.

Another common and inappropriate reason for not studying is illness. Commonly, when we see a singer with laryngitis in our medical offices and determine that he or she may proceed cautiously with a performance provided other vocal activities are limited, the singer will

3

often cancel his or her voice lessons. The weak, sick or injured singer's voice needs supervision of technique more than ever. Singing lessons under such circumstances may be short and directed, toward assuring that the singer's technique has remained excellent despite deficits in auditory feedback (from "stuffy ears" caused by a cold, for example). Vocal nodules are also not a reason to stop singing lessons, although they may be a good reason to stop public performance. Supervised, correct singing does not cause vocal nodules; and, in the author's (RTS) voice center, we use singing lessons routinely in association with speaking voice therapy in the treatment of vocal nodules and other benign vocal fold masses.

A third common (and equally invalid) reason for not studying is vocal experience. Even premier singers in the best opera companies continue to study and to have an objective expert monitor their vocal techniques. Unfortunately, when they do not, the public usually becomes aware of it before long; and sometimes this shortsightedness leads to vocal injuries that require medical or surgical care. None of us is so experienced or so expert as to be able to abandon vocal study altogether. Certainly, the young artist who is in the first years of touring will find it difficult to continue voice lessons, and may underestimate their importance since he or she is already "successful"; but this shortsightedness eventually causes trouble in most cases.

4

Don't recognize technical problems in your singing voice

Technical errors in voices may be the primary cause of a medical voice complaint or may develop secondarily as a result of a singer's efforts to compensate for voice disturbance from another cause.

Singing should not hurt the throat. If, at the end of a voice lesson, a singer is tired and aches a bit in his or her lower back or abdomen, that is usually not a problem. However, if pain occurs in neck, throat or larynx, that may be a danger signal. Most often, it is caused by excessive tension in the neck and tongue that is not necessary for good singing and may be unhealthy for the voice, even leading to vocal nodules or other vocal fold pathology. Early in training, a little discomfort in the neck is not uncommon as a singer's bad technique is being corrected; but it should become progressively better and disappear during the course of training.

Hoarseness following voice lessons is also another danger signal. Hoarseness usually is caused by damage on the delicate leading edges of the vocal folds. It does not ordinarily occur after proper singing. If it occurs consistently following voice lessons, this maybe an important warning.

The number of years a performer has been training his or her voice may be a fair index of vocal proficiency. A person who has studied voice for one or two years is somewhat more likely to have gross technical difficulties than someone who has been studying for 20 years. However, if training has been intermittent or discontinued, technical problems are common even among experienced singers.

In addition, methods of technical voice use vary among voice teachers. Hence, a student who has had many teachers in a relatively brief period of time commonly has numerous technical insecurities or deficiencies that may be responsible for vocal dysfunction. This is especially true if the singer has changed to a new teacher within the preceding year. The physician must be careful not to criticize the patient's current voice teacher in such circumstances. It often takes years of expert instruction to correct bad habits.

5

Speak as you would never dare to sing

Singers always should use their voices as if their careers depended on them – in speech or in song – because they do. Most trained singers are very careful about the way they use their voices during singing. The amount of voice use and training also affects voice. They support their tones, they do not sing too loudly, they are fussy about room conditions such as temperature, humidity and acoustics, and they are sensitive to every nuance. Yet, too often all of this excellent technique is forgotten as soon as the singer begins to speak. Unfortunately, few singers have formal training in the use of the speaking voice; and most of us do not carry over the techniques of support and breath control from our singing training to our speaking without additional instruction. Often, when a singer is hoarse on the morning after a performance, the hoarseness is due not to the singing, but to the backstage greetings and post-performance celebrations. Vocal injury from speaking voice abuse is reflected in the singing voice.

Voice abuse such as yelling is an extremely common source of hoarseness, vocal weakness, pain, and other complaints. In some cases, voice abuse can even create structural problems such as vocal nodules, cysts, and polyps.

If voice abuse is caused by speaking, treatment should be provided by a licensed certified speech language pathologist in the United States or by a phoniatrist in many other countries. Training the speaking voice benefits singers greatly not only by improving speech but also by helping singing technique indirectly. Specialized singing training also may be helpful to many voice professionals who are not singers, and it is invaluable for patients who are singers. Voice professionals include not only actors and media stars, but also teachers, secretaries, clergy, lawyers, sales people and anyone else whose work (or serious association) would be harmed by voice impairment.

Initial singing training teaches relaxation techniques, develops muscle strength, and should be symbiotic with standard voice therapy. Abuse of the voice during singing is an even more complex problem that can be addressed by expert singing teachers (technique) and voice coaches (repertoire and style). It is always possible to do the "wrong thing" (like screaming on stage) the right way. The singer just needs to master the necessary craft BEFORE getting into trouble and ending up in our medical offices.

6

Wear yourself out

Have you ever wondered why singers get sick before performances? Most people think it is because singers are all hypochondriacs; but that is rarely the case. Ordinarily, a singer practices scales for half an hour or an hour daily and may sing for another two or three hours during the course of the day. However, preceding performances, the singer may rehearse twelve or fourteen hours a day for two or three weeks, in a strange city with unfamiliar environmental conditions, potential allergens, and may be sleeping poorly in a strange hotel bed. At these times, singers are under maximum physical and emotional stress. The voice is a finely tuned instrument. The body needs sleep, food (a reasonably well balanced diet), and lots of fluids in order to maintain that fine tuning. When we stay up too late, our eyes get "bloodshot" and start to burn. Similar changes in mucosal lubrication and irritability occur throughout the vocal tract. When we wear ourselves out, we interfere with the body's ability to repair, replenish, and balance the components of our vocal mechanisms. Consciously recognizing this scenario often allows singers to avoid its pitfalls. Learning roles in advance, staying well hydrated, arriving in a city a day or two before rehearsals begin to adjust to the climate (especially in cities at high altitude), and avoiding extraneous activities that tire the voice or interfere with rest are often helpful and sufficient to avoid problems.

7

Sing the wrong music

There are many different types of performances and auditions that a singer will encounter during his or her career. All singers would love to perform at the highest level at all times, but that is not a realistic goal. There will be periods when you are injured or not in the best health. As your own advocate, you must decide the importance of each event in achieving your overall professional goals.

At one time or another, all of us have a tendency to be dissatisfied with the limitations of our voices. Baritones want to be tenors, lyric sopranos want to be "high coloraturas", etc. Most commonly, young singers want to sound older than their years. Attempts to make the voice something that it is not, or that it is not yet, often stress the voice and may produce significant harm. Unfortunately, occasionally young singers are encouraged to sing inappropriate material by music school faculty in order to fill needed roles in opera or show music productions, or to enhance the apparent maturity of a recital. All of us must resist the temptation to stretch voices beyond their proper limits, choosing repertoire with the greatest of care.

8

Sing in noise

In a sense, we nearly always sing in noisy environments. Singers and instrumentalists need to be made more aware of the hazards of noise exposure and find ways to avoid or reduce its effects whenever possible. Classical singers learn to accommodate the noise and to "balance" their voices. When they are accompanied by a piano, this is relatively easy, so long as the singer has an opportunity to "gauge" the performance hall in advance. In assessing the room, the singer (or speaker) should investigate acoustics, type of microphones available, room temperature, availability of water, and presence or absence of a stage manager, among other factors. However, even well-trained, young, classical singers may have this training break down in specific circumstances such as their first experience singing with (or against) a large orchestra, in their first outdoor performances, and in other situations in which auditory feedback is impaired. Classical singers are trained to compensate for such problems by learning to monitor their performance with proprioceptive feedback (by feel) rather than auditory feedback (by ear). Popular singers are required to sing in the presence of extreme noise produced by electrical instruments and exuberant audiences. Their salvation is a device called a "monitor speaker" which may be a speaker or an in-the-ear device. This directs the voice back to the singer, so that one's own voice can be heard. Unfortunately, monitor speakers are expensive, and they often are controlled by a well-trained "sound man" who may not want to make them loud enough for the singer to hear (because of artistic reasons or technical problems such as feedback).

Because of cost, many singing students who perform in popular bands in order to earn money do not invest in monitor speakers. These are the people who need them most. Singers who perform music of this sort should be encouraged strongly to purchase monitors, and to have them adjusted so that they can hear them comfortably.

9

Speak in noise

The "Lombard Effect" is the tendency to speak more loudly in the presence of background noise. At parties, we shout. Under these circumstances, we are rarely aware of good abdominal support and voice conservation techniques. Such abuse can wreak havoc on a voice, particularly when it is already tired after an evening of singing performance. Singers who perform a series of concerts tend to be more aware of post-performance voice conservation than others. However, any singer should protect the voice at all times as if the greatest opportunity of his/her career were going to come unexpectedly tomorrow. Sometimes it does. Party rooms are not the only environments that predispose to speaking louder than we realize. Cars and airplanes are also particularly noisy. Airplane travel compounds the problem with the addition of low humidity, which dehydrates the singer. Ideally, singers should study speaking technique and should be aware of their vocal and auditory environments constantly, and they should protect themselves accordingly. In short order, this behavior becomes second nature.

10

Conduct

Amateur choral conducting is especially hazardous to singers unless the singer is trained well in conducting technique. Many singers conduct in order to earn money while they are waiting to be "discovered." Unfortunately, most such musicians have limited formal training in conducting, and usually they are relegated to conducting amateur choirs. Amateur groups are much more vocally taxing to a conductor than groups composed of trained singers. Most singers haven't had enough conducting expertise to be able to conduct a well-paced rehearsal while maintaining minimal body motion, good balance, and excellent vocal technique. Intermittently, they end up singing soprano, alto, tenor, and bass at volumes louder than the entire ensemble. Singers who choose conducting as a vocation should develop specific, conscious techniques to preserve their voices during rehearsals; and they should make the effort to study conducting formally. Conducting can certainly be done safely; but, like singing, it requires skill. Hoarseness in a conductor following rehearsals is an important warning. Hoarseness in the chorus singers is also an indication of faulty conducting technique!

Choirs are among our noisiest environments. An enthusiastic choral conductor can often get singers to sing more loudly than they would ever sing alone in their living rooms. Young professional singers often encounter difficulty singing in choral environments, particularly if they are hired as part of a professional quartet affiliated with an amateur (church) choir. Such singers often feel that part of their responsibility is to lead the section; and this is often interpreted as singing louder than the section. We advise our patients who are choir members as follows:

Sing as if you are giving a voice lesson to the person standing on each side of you, and as if there is a microphone immediately in front of you that is recording your choral singing for your voice teacher.

This approach usually not only solves the problem, but also results in a better choral sound.

11

Teach voice

Voice teaching can be hazardous to your vocal health. Like conducting, it can certainly be done safely, but it requires skill and thought. Most voice teachers teach seated at a piano on a bench with no back support and often incapable of height adjustment. Late in a long, hard day, the slouching posture that often results is not conducive to maintenance of optimal abdominal and back support for the singing that teachers often used to model for their children. Often, we also teach with students continuously positioned to our right or left. This may require the teacher to turn his or her neck at a particularly sharp angle, especially when teaching with an upright piano in a small studio. Teachers also have a tendency to demonstrate vocal materials in their students' ranges, rather than their own. If a singing teacher is hoarse or has neck discomfort, or if soft singing control deteriorates at the end of the day (assuming the teacher warms up before beginning voice lessons and cools down often), voice abuse should be suspected. Helpful modifications include teaching with a grand piano, sitting slightly sideways on the piano bench, or alternating student position to the right and left of the piano to facilitate better neck alignment. Retaining an accompanist so that the teacher can stand rather than teach from behind the piano, and many other helpful modifications are possible. Shortening voice lessons slightly is also recommended highly. Singing teachers typically teach a 60-minute hour (as opposed to the 50-minute hour used by speech pathologists to leave time for chart documentation). Then, teachers may see students for hours with no vocal break. Using a 50 or even 55-minute hour with 5 or 10 minutes of vocal rest between each lesson and time for a few minutes of gentle cool down exercises a few times a day can make a great difference in a singing teacher's vocal health and longevity. However, the first and most important step is for the voice teacher to recognize the studio as a potentially hazardous area to the voice and become aware of personal vocal behavior.

12

Smoke

The effects of tobacco smoke on the vocal folds have been known for many years.[1] Smoking not only causes chronic irritation, but it can also result in microscopic alterations in the vocal fold epithelium. The epithelial cells change their appearance, becoming increasingly different from normal epithelial cells. Eventually, they begin to pile up on each other, rather than lining up in an orderly fashion. Then they escape normal homeostatic controls, growing rapidly without restraint and invading surrounding tissues. This drastic change is called squamous cell carcinoma, or cancer of the larynx. Anyone concerned about the health of his or her voice should not smoke.

It is astonishing to most of us involved with voice care that so many singers still use tobacco. The adverse effects of tobacco smoke are well documented and incontestable. In addition to its long-term health consequences, such as cancer of the larynx, lung cancer, emphysema, blood vessel disease, and other major illnesses, smoke has immediate, deleterious effects on the larynx and the linings of the respiratory tract. It produces inflammation (redness and swelling) that alters the vocal folds and lungs themselves. If smokers who have accommodated to these abnormalities have any doubt that they occur, they need only ask non-smoking singers who are forced to perform in smoky environments. Heavy smoking also decreases respiratory function over time, undermining the power source of the voice. The argument that "there have been many great singers who smoke" is a bad one. A singer has a responsibility to optimize his/her own instrument – to be as good a singer as he or she possibly can be. While some people can adapt fairly well for many years to the chronic irritation of tobacco smoke, their laryngeal and respiratory condition is never as good as it would be without the effects of smoke. This is true even if they smoke through a Hookah, although Hookahs help filter and cool tobacco, probably rendering it less irritating than smoke inhaled directly from cigarettes.

Some vocalists are required to perform in smoke-filled environments and may suffer the same effects as smokers themselves. In some theaters, it is possible to place fans upstage or direct the ventilation system so as to create a gentle draft towards the audience, clearing the smoke away from the stage. Smoke eaters installed in some theaters are also helpful. Exposure to environmental tobacco smoke, also called secondhand smoke, is the passive inhalation of tobacco smoke from environmental sources, such as smoke given off by pipes, cigars, and cigarettes or the smoke exhaled from the lungs of smokers and inhaled by other people. This passive smoke contains a mixture of thousands of chemicals, some of which are known to cause cancer. The National Institutes of Health (NIH) lists environmental tobacco smoke as a known carcinogen, and the more you are exposed to secondhand smoke, the greater your risk.[1]

Pipe smoke and cigar smoke have the same effects as cigarette smoke, but often to a lesser degree as they are not intentionally inhaled routinely. However, smokeless or chewing tobacco is highly addictive, and users who dip eight to ten times a day may have the same nicotine exposure as those who smoke one to two packs of cigarettes per day. Smokeless tobacco has been associated with gingivitis, cheek carcinoma, and cancer of the larynx and hypopharynx. The radiation or surgical excision of the tongue or floor of mouth required to treat these cancers certainly can end a singing career.

Marijuana smoke is particularly harsh, hot and unfiltered; and its content is unregulated and unpredictable in most locales. In addition, it may alter sensorium, interfering with fine motor control and the intellectual awareness intrinsic to good, safe singing. Its use should be avoided in serious singers. However, like cigarette smoking, the use of marijuana probably will not be eliminated entirely even among professional singers. If used at all, marijuana should at least be smoked through a water pipe which partially filters and cools the smoke.

References

1. US Dept of Health and Human Services, Public Health Service, National Toxicology Program (NTP). Report on Carcinogens. 12th ed. Research Triangle Park, NC: NTP; 2011.

13

Drink alcohol

Alcohol poses several problems for the singer. First, it is a vasodilator. That is, it opens up blood vessels (including those in the larynx (or voice box)), and alters mucosal secretions which are so important to singing. Second, it alters awareness and fine motor control, even after consumption of very small amounts. Voice training is directed toward establishing meticulous control over the many muscles required for singing, through instantaneous self-assessment and adjustment. Alcohol is terrific at undermining all those years in the studio.

From a practical point of view, very small amounts of alcohol in people who are accustomed to drinking do not seem to pose a major problem. For example, a singer who routinely has a glass of wine with dinner need not *necessarily* alter this daily routine a few hours before performance. However, larger amounts may be harmful to a performer even in people who consume alcoholic beverages regularly. Singers who are not accustomed to drinking routinely should be particularly careful to avoid alcohol on the day of a performance. In addition to the intoxicating and vasodilating effects, many people have mild allergies to certain alcoholic beverages. These are most frequently manifested as nasal congestion and clear nasal discharge and are seen most commonly following ingestion of beverages that contain yeast (beer) and certain varieties of grapes (wines). For this reason, on the day of a performance, singers should not consume beverages with which they have no experience so that they do not accidentally initiate an allergic response.

14

Take "recreational" drugs

Like alcohol, most street drugs alter sensorium. In singers, the decreased awareness and impairment of accurate analytic abilities undermine good vocal technique. They not only prevent a singer from recognizing the need to make the instantaneous modifications that are intrinsic to good singing, but some street drugs also interfere with reaction time and motor control directly, impairing the ability to make the adjustments even when the need is recognized. In some cases, they may also decrease feeling (particularly narcotics) and allow a singer to injure himself/herself without feeling pain. This can result in serious or permanent vocal fold damage as the singer continues to use his or her voice, perhaps remaining oblivious to the vocal problem until the next day. Certain street drugs, particularly "uppers," also may cause a tremor that can be heard in the singing voice. In addition, the exact composition of street drugs is rarely known, and various compounds added by dealers have serious health implications. For instance, "designer drugs" have caused complications ranging from complete rigidity of all muscles in some users, to death in others.

15

Eat, drink, and be merry

Everyone enjoys the good life. Nevertheless, singers must remember that they are athletes constantly in training. Many successful singers are gregarious, verbal, and orally oriented. They are also famished after a hard evening's performance. Excessive eating and "partying" may be hazardous, especially late in the evening. It predisposes to reflux laryngitis and to weight gain. Obesity is as unhealthy for singers as it is for any other athlete. It also may interfere with abdominal and respiratory support, predisposing to improper singing technique. The singer also must be especially wary of speaking in noisy restaurants and party situations after alcohol consumption. A full stomach impairing support, mild (or more than mild) intoxication dulling awareness, and loud background noise predisposing to excessive speaking volume can wreak havoc on a voice. Such circumstances often result in hoarseness the morning after a performance that was sung flawlessly; and sometimes they result in potential catastrophe, such as vocal hemorrhage.

16

Prescribe your own medicines

After reading from the internet for an hour or two, too many singers think that they know as much about medicine as their laryngologists; and who wants to spend all that money going to the doctor anyway? While it is certainly true that the experienced singer who has consulted regularly with an expert laryngologist often recognizes the symptoms of illness and knows the usual treatments; prescribing for one's self can be dangerous. For the most part, medicines are chemicals. In the right doses at the right times, they may work miracles. However, in the wrong doses, for the wrong duration, at the wrong time, or in the wrong person, they may be harmful or even fatal. Borrowing medications from a colleague is especially hazardous, as they may contain allergenic components of which neither singer is unaware. Certain types of drugs are abused with particular frequency.

Antibiotics should be used only for specific bacterial infections. They do not cure viruses, such as the ones that cause the common cold. There are many different kinds of antibiotics, some of which are totally ineffective against certain kinds of bacteria. For example, Penicillin may work well on most cases of strep throat; but if the bacterial infection is caused by staphylococcus rather than streptococcus, Penicillin is often not helpful. In fact, if the dose is too low or the medication is not taken long enough, an inappropriate antibiotic can even turn an easily curable infection into a resistant infection requiring prolonged, expensive medication, or even hospitalization.

Steroids, such as Prednisone, decrease inflammation and may improve singing by removing fluid from "boggy" vocal folds. However, they also impair the body's ability to respond to infection. They should be used only under specific circumstances, in appropriate doses, and often in combination with antibiotics. The judgment on their advisability should rarely be made without visualization of the vocal folds by an expert physician.

Antihistamines counteract allergy symptoms. However, they also are very effective "drying" agents for the upper respiratory tract. They may greatly decrease or thicken vocal fold lubrication, resulting in a dry "tickle" and cough. They also are often combined with decongestants that can sometimes produce tremor. Antihistamines should be used in singers only for very specific indications, and virtually never given for the first time immediately before performance.

Diuretics are water pills often misused to decrease premenstrual fluid retention. Unfortunately, they do not diurese fluid bound to protein, as it occurs in the vocal folds. They do effectively diurese free fluid, such as that needed for lubrication of the vocal fold edges. Therefore, in a singer who has trouble with her voice in the immediate premenstrual period, they may actually make things worse by impairing surface lubrication without mitigating the "boggy" vocal folds.

Aspirin seems like a safe enough medication to use on your own. Actually, it has many potentially serious side effects in the singer and should almost never be used if there is an alternative. Of greatest importance is its tendency to cause bleeding. Aspirin is used as an anticoagulant in patients with heart and blood vessel disease. Any singer who requires surgery, laryngeal or non-laryngeal, must inform their surgeon that he or she is taking aspirin. Aspirin and aspirin containing products must be stopped 7–10 days preoperatively (depending on the surgeon), in order to prevent untoward intraoperative and postoperative complications (bleeding). Moreover, aspirin predisposes the singer to vocal fold hemorrhage especially when used for menstrual cramps, because the

25

premenstrual hormonal environment results in capillary fragility and increased bleeding tendency even without the added drug effect; and cramps may interfere with effective support. The combination can be disastrous.

 Similar caveats hold true for other medications including many over-the-counter and some alternative/complementary preparations. For every good therapeutic effect, there are numerous potential bad side effects. Medicines are best administered under medical supervision. See your doctor.

17

Don't recognize the risks of taking complementary and alternative remedies

Over the past couple of decades, the medical community has seen a dramatic increase in the number of individuals using alternative/complementary medication in the form of herbs and dietary supplements. Some complementary/alternative medicine (CAM) products including herbal preparations are useful and some have no proven efficacy. Recommended dosages of these products are not agreed upon universally and they are not regulated by the FDA (Federal Drug Administration) in the United States or by federal agencies in most other countries. Many individuals make the mistake of equating "natural" with safe and effective. Singers and all voice users must be aware that many CAMs used commonly have potential side effects, including diuretic, hormonal and anticoagulation action. Any and all ingested products have potential for adverse reactions.

Singers and all patients should be encouraged not to use these products indiscriminately and should consult their physician and/or laryngologist before using.

Herbal Medications	Risks Associated with Use
Echinacea	Can be immunosuppressive
Garlic & Ginger	Anticoagulation activity
Melatonin	Has hormonal activity and can also cause immune dysregulation
Vitamin E	Taken in megadoses (4000 IU or greater), it has anticoagulation activity (anti-platelet)
Ginkgo	Bleeding, GI upset, headache, palpitations
St. John's Wort	Insomnia, anxiety, GI upset, vivid dreams, fatigue, photosensitivity, intermenstrual ("breakthrough") bleeding
Ginseng	Agitation, insomnia, nervousness
Aloe	GI upset, heart disturbances, low blood sugar levels

18

Only see your doctor when you're desperate

Doctors are expensive, but so is loss of your voice. In fact, in many cities, a visit to a laryngologist costs less than a voice lesson. The longer a singer waits before visiting a doctor, the worse his or her condition might be. Moreover, the more time between the doctor visit and a performance commitment, the better the chances of effective medical care and safe singing. When the singer starts to feel "sick" on Sunday or Monday and has major singing commitments on Friday, it simply doesn't pay to wait until Thursday and risk having to cancel the concert or sing in ill health. Frequently, the physician will have recently seen many people with the same symptoms (upper respiratory infection (URI), viruses, GI infections, the flu, and others), and will know immediately how to treat the condition to prevent it from getting worse. Early or preventive care saves a lot of wear and tear on your voice (and on your doctor).

19

Choose the wrong doctor

Not all doctors are voice specialists. It is exceedingly difficult for a lay person to know how to judge whether the doctor he or she picks is the right physician for him or her. Not even all ear, nose, and throat specialists may be presumed to be experts on care of the singing voice. The first ear, nose, and throat text book with a chapter on care of the professional voice wasn't released until 1986;[1] and the first medical text book on the subject wasn't published until 1991.[2] In fact, the subject of care for the professional voice users is relatively new in physician training. Not all of the residency programs in the United States teach it at all. However, over the past two decades, fellowship training in laryngology has been created with a focus on voice care. Fortunately, in recent years, many more otolaryngologists have become interested in voice and have attended courses at Academy meetings, The Voice Foundation's Annual Symposium: Care of the Professional Voice and other such educational programs. It is important for singers to be as well educated as possible about all aspects of the voice and its maladies, not only so they may help a good laryngologist reach an expeditious and correct diagnosis, but also so that they can choose a good doctor and know when their doctor's advice doesn't make sense.

References

1. Sataloff, R.T. The Professional Voice. In: Cummings, C.W., Frederickson, J.M., Harker, L.A., Krause, C.J., Schuller, D.E. (Eds) *Otolaryngology-Head and Neck Surgery*. St. Louis, MO: C.V. Mosby; 1986:2029–2056.

2. Sataloff, R.T. *Professional Voice: The Science and Art of Clinical Care*, Third Edition. San Diego, CA: Plural Publishing, Inc.; 2005.

20

Choose the wrong voice teacher

If defining a good laryngologist seems hard, then defining a good voice teacher approaches the impossible. This is obviously a challenge for singing students. However, it also is a problem for laryngologists who often ask us how to find a good voice teacher for their patients. There will be no attempt to cover this challenging and controversial subject fully in this chapter. This topic has inspired hundreds of articles and books, as well as endless research. However, from a medical point of view (leaving my (RTS) biases as a singing teacher aside as much as possible), a few general observations may be helpful. To a great degree, vocal training consists of muscle development and coordination. Once muscles are shaped and contoured, they maintain their shape for many years. For example, people in their eighties seen on the beach in the summer still have bulging biceps from exercises they have not performed for 30 or 40 years. Consequently, the importance of expert training for the beginner cannot be over emphasized. There is often a tendency to send the young singer to "the teacher down the street" for a few years or to the graduate teaching assistant to find out whether the student has any real talent. While the teacher down the street or the graduate student *might* turn out to be an excellent teacher, inadequate investigation of his or her capabilities is common for the student who is "only a beginner." There is no point in a singer's vocal training at which expert teaching is more important, or at which there is a potential for a profound and irreversible effect on the vocal mechanism. Unfortunately, some of the blame for this situation rests with expert teachers who often make themselves unavailable not only to pop singers, but also to beginners. While we all recognize the exigencies and demands of a busy teaching career, the relative paucity of top flight teachers for beginners should be a matter of greater concern and action within the singing teacher community.

Now, what is an excellent voice teacher? At a bare minimum, the student may have a few reasonable expectations of what should and should not happen during the course of vocal training.

Abdominal and back muscle strength and breathing ability should improve. These functions form the power source of the singing voice, our so-called "support." Although there are many valid approaches to teaching breathing and support, the development of this component of the vocal mechanism is essential.

The voice should improve, but not necessarily immediately. Learning to sing may take time. Often, as a singer abandons "bad habits," the voice actually sounds worse for a time while strength is being developed in appropriate muscles. However, over a period of many months, note by note improvement in vocal quality and ease should be expected.

If the singer experiences discomfort while singing and his/her teacher says that everything is "fine," it is reasonable for the singer to be concerned. Seeking a "second opinion" from another voice teacher or specialist may be warranted. People obtain second opinions with regard to their medical care all the time, without causing offense to their primary physician. Voice teachers often are more sensitive than they should be, considering this as an insult rather than an opportunity to obtain additional professional input to help their students.

Good teachers generally are able to avoid vocal trauma of the magnitude necessary to cause hoarseness. Hoarseness can arise if the singer's voice teacher is unable to recognize and correct "pushed" or "forced" sound or if the teacher allows the singer to sing for unreasonably long periods of time (the time varies with the level of expertise). Correcting issues with hoarseness requires a very slow training process, vocalizing with only a few notes for short lessons while building up vocal strength and skill, but there is virtually always a way to avoid it unless there is an underlying medical problem. Naturally, it is incumbent upon the singing student to be patient and cooperate with a good teacher's method, even if vocal progress seems slower than the student would like.

It is not reasonable for a singer to expect that even a singing teacher who is known to be superb will be right for all singers. We all have different personalities, and only the very best teachers in any field can alter their approaches drastically enough to communicate with equal facility with all students. It is certainly best to find a teacher who has had great and consistent success; but after a trial, if the teacher and student are not communicating effectively and making progress, discussions of referral to another voice teacher at least for evaluation and possibly for training are reasonable. Most good voice teachers are willing to discuss and consider this possibility, and even to make the referral.

Beware of the voice teacher who is too secretive. Most good teachers have no compunction about having their lessons observed occasionally, about having their students listened to under proper circumstances, and about having them evaluated by a qualified laryngologist. The teacher who insists on isolating his/her students, discourages medical consultation, and discourages education about the voice from other sources (books, pedagogy courses, articles) should be scrutinized with great skepticism.

21

Choose the wrong schedule

Damage can be caused by over-taxing the voice through excessive travel, insufficient preparation, repertoire demands, and too many concerts. However, the broader exposure of career schedules also should be considered. Voices mature at different rates. If a singer plans at 18 to make his Metropolitan Opera debut as Rigoletto at the age of 23, he may push vocal training and over-schedule performance commitments in a self-imposed five-year schedule. When we try to rush nature, the body and voice frequently rebel. Each singer needs to be honest with him- or herself and seek the advice of experienced teachers and coaches. A serious singer's performance plan may span more than a decade. However, conservative, slow progression and development with appropriate repertoire predispose to strong, healthy, durable voices. Impatience, bad advice, and self-deception predispose to an early career change.

22

Choose the wrong career

Although it sounds obvious to say that not everyone is destined to be a professional singer, a few evenings in concert halls and community opera houses confirm that it is not so obvious, at least to some singers. Not everyone is destined to be the kind of singer he or she aspires to be. The lyric tenor determined to sing *Siegfried*, the baritone determined to sing tenor, the singer with a light, pleasant popular voice determined to sing grand opera, and other singers with inaccurate self-perception frequently damage not only their egos, but also their larynges. In fact, this author (RTS) believes virtually everyone can sing. Moreover, everyone can sing better with training than without. A singer who chooses a career for which his or her voice is not suited may damage the voice and potentially abandon an equally gratifying but attainable career in performance or in something else with vocal performance as an avocation.

Self-assessment is difficult for anyone in any field. It is often helpful for the serious-minded young singer who has had a few years of training to sing for a few unbiased masters in the area of his or her interest. This is often accomplished most effectively with people who do not know the singer or his/her family, and perhaps who live in another city. For example, for a young singer with serious operatic aspirations, a trip to New York to audition for major conductors, teachers, or agents, or a few weeks at an opera camp or summer music camp, may provide the kind of feedback needed. Sometimes the assessments are encouraging, and sometimes they hurt; but an honest, accurate evaluation of a singer's voice and its best potential is invaluable in planning an appropriate career. Devoting one's energies toward pursuit of a career for which one is physically and vocally ill-suited is a nearly certain road to a short career.

23

Choose the wrong "day job"

Frequently, singers have non-musical jobs to support themselves while pursuing their singing careers. As discussed earlier, a singer should not treat his or her speaking voice with any less care and skill than his or her singing voice, and this axiom should be considered when taking a non-musical job. Jobs such as waitressing in crowded, noisy restaurants can cause one to increase vocal intensity, leading to unsafe volumes, abusive behaviors, and potentially serious vocal fold pathology. It is also difficult to support well while carrying trays and leaning over tables to be heard over noise. Other jobs that require extensive speaking (including teaching) may cause voice problems that affect singing.

A singer should suspect voice abuse when he or she experiences vocal fatigue and hoarseness at the end of the work day or week, and should be evaluated by a laryngologist. Working with a singing voice specialist and speech language pathologist can help to improve vocal hygiene and provide the singers with the skills to optimize voice use even under adverse circumstances. However, when job options with fewer vocal demands are viable, they should be considered seriously. Even if you are a data entry clerk, try not to be a typical, chatty singer who spends all day socializing with people over computer noise!

24

Choose the wrong singing voice specialist

A singing voice specialist (SVS) is a singing voice teacher trained to work with injured or abused voices. There are no formal training programs, and the singer should be aware of potential variations of training and expertise in this field. The SVS is usually part of a voice team and works closely with a laryngologist and speech language pathologist or phoniatrist in the care of the voice patient. A joint committee of The American Speech-Language-Hearing Association (ASHA) and National Association of Teachers of Singing (NATS) has compiled a list of professional SVSs who have undergone some degree of interdisciplinary training in this field.[1] Basic, core knowledge that the SVS should acquire has been proposed.

During evaluation with an SVS, the singer is asked about abusive habits, typical performance environments, career goals, and prior training. The singer's stance/posture, breath, support, and positioning of the larynx, tongue, jaw, and face are evaluated. The degree to which abnormalities can be corrected quickly with cues is assessed. Exercises are given to the singer to optimize support and technique and decrease potentially dangerous excessive tension. The frequency and duration of sessions with the SVS depend on the needs of the singer and the laryngologist's advice.

References

1. Sataloff, R.T., Baroody, M.M., Emerich, K.A., Carroll, L.M. The Singing Voice Specialist. In: Sataloff, R.T. *Professional Voice: The Science and Art of Clinical Care.* Third edition. San Diego, CA: Plural Publishing, Inc.; 2005: 1021–1039.

Choose the wrong speech-language pathologist

A speech-language pathologist (SLP) receives training in the treatment of a variety of communication and swallowing disorders. Frequently, little time is devoted to voice disorders during education, and typically a SLP who is interested in voice therapy seeks additional training following completion of his or her training program. A singer must be aware of these variations. There is no standardized credentialing process for a SLP with a focus on voice. Commonly, a SLP specializing in voice therapy is part of voice team that conducts a multidisciplinary approach to voice evaluation and treatment. It is important for a singer to choose a SLP who is trained to treat singers and voice disorders.

During a voice evaluation, a singer may be asked to complete the Voice Handicap Index (VHI)[1] to quantify the degree of vocal impairment. This is a questionnaire that lets health care professionals know how a voice disorder is affecting the life of the specific patient under evaluation. Evaluation includes perceptual assessment of the voice, objective voice evaluation, and laryngeal examination. The physician and SLP devise a treatment plan using the information from the examination and history. Typically during voice therapy, a SLP will educate the singer about voice disorders and review examination findings. The process of voice therapy, treatment goals, and vocal hygiene are discussed. Duration and frequency of therapy are dependent on the severity of the vocal dysfunction and on the patient's ability to modify vocal behaviors and sustain the changes.

References

1. Jacobson, B.H., Johnson, A., Grywalski, C., et al. The Voice Handicap Index (VHI): development and validation. *Am J Speech-Lang Pathol.* 1997; 6:66–70.

Don't recognize that gastrointestinal (GI) disorders commonly cause voice complaints

Gastroesophageal reflux can cause laryngitis. This is called laryngopharyngeal reflux (LPR). In LPR, stomach acid refluxes into the throat, allowing droplets of the irritating gastric juices to come in contact with the vocal folds and even be aspirated into the lungs. Reflux may occur with or without a hiatal hernia. Common symptoms are hoarseness, prolonged vocal warm-up time, bad breath, sensation of a lump in the throat, chronic sore throat, cough, and a dry or coated mouth. Typical heartburn is frequently absent. Lifestyle changes such as quitting smoking and losing weight, avoiding medications and supplements that irritate the esophageal lining, reducing the meal size and acidity, and reducing the quantity of fluids consumed can reduce reflux symptoms in some people. Over time, uncontrolled reflux may cause cancer of the esophagus and larynx. LPR should be treated conscientiously. Laryngeal examination usually reveals a bright red, often slightly swollen appearance of the mucosa overlying the arytenoid cartilages at the back of the larynx, which helps establish the diagnosis. The mainstays of treatment are diet modification, elevation of the head of the bed in some patients, use of antacid medications, and avoidance of food for three or four hours before going to sleep. Avoidance of alcohol and coffee is beneficial. Medications that often block acid secretion are essential, including H2-blockers and proton pump inhibitors. In some cases, surgery to repair the lower esophageal sphincter and cure the reflux may be more appropriate than lifelong medical management.

Eating a full meal before a singing or speaking engagement may interfere with the abdominal support and may aggravate upright reflux of gastric juice during abdominal muscle contraction. Highly spiced or acidic foods may cause mucosal irritation and also aggravate reflux laryngitis. Coffee and other beverages containing caffeine aggravate gastric reflux and may promote dehydration and/or alter secretions and necessitate frequent throat clearing in some people. Fad diets, especially rapid weight reduction diets, are notorious for causing voice problems. Some diets (such as low-acid) may help patients with reflux.

Any condition that alters function, such as muscle spasm, constipation or diarrhea, and pregnancy may interfere with support and may result in voice complaint. GI symptoms may accompany infection, anxiety, various gastrointestinal diseases, and other maladies.

Suggested Reading

Sataloff, R.T., Katz, P.O., Sataloff, D.M. and Hawkshaw, M.J. *Reflux Laryngitis and Related Disorders*, Fourth Edition. San Diego, CA: Plural Publishing, Inc.; 2013.

Koufman, J., Stern, J. and Bauer, M. *Dropping Acid: The Reflux Diet Cookbook & Cure*. New York, NY: The Reflux Cookbooks, LLC; 2010.

Aviv, E. J. *Killing Me Softly From Inside: The Mysteries & Dangers of Acid Reflux and its Connection to America's Fastest Growing Cancer with a Diet that May Save Your Life*. New York, NY: CNB Productions LLC; 2014.

27

Neglect treating your allergies

Allergies, even if mild, can affect a singer's voice. Changes in the mucosa and secretions can affect the nose and larynx. These changes can be seasonal or year round depending upon the trigger. Allergy testing and evaluation may be helpful for management and avoidance of allergens.

Frequently, oral medications used to treat allergy can have unfavorable side effects, which is why it is important to inform your allergist that you are a singer. For example, some of the more commonly prescribed and over-the-counter medications (Allegra (fexofenadine Hcl) (Sanofi-Aventis, Paris, France), Zyrtec (cetirizine) (McNeil-PPC, Inc., Fort Washington, PA), Claritin (loratadine) (Merck Sharp & Dohme Corp., Whitehouse Station, NJ), and other antihistamines, including Benadryl (diphenhydramine) (McNeil-PPC, Inc., Fort Washington, PA) can be drying and particularly irritating to singers. Nasal steroid sprays (Nasonex (mometasone furoate monohydrate) (Merck Sharp & Dohme Corp., Whitehouse Station, NJ), Flonase (fluticasone propionate) (GlaxoSmithKline, Brentford, UK) may be beneficial if used correctly. Steroid sprays only act topically, avoiding systemic effects found in oral steroid use, and they avoid having the medication reach the larynx where it can cause irritation. Saline gels, sprays, and irrigations are also helpful in treating nasal dryness. If an acute allergic flair develops, oral steroid therapy may be helpful to maximize voice quality and minimize symptoms, but this is not a long-term solution.

Following identification of allergens, environmental modification may be helpful. For example, antiallergenic bed and pillow covers are helpful in those allergic to dust mites. However, they may not be practical for touring singers who spend 200 nights a year in a hotel rooms. Moreover, allergies vary between locations, and a singer's allergies may be more problematic depending on the location. One of the more favorable treatments for singers is immunotherapy (shots), as it lacks some of the side effects discussed above. During treatment, injections of increasing concentrations of identified allergens are administered to decrease the allergic response. This treatment is not appropriate for all patients. Furthermore, if a singer typically spends time in two locations (e.g. Philadelphia in the winter and Spoleto in the summer) shots must be designed to treat allergies from both locales.

28

Neglect treating your asthma

Breathing is an important component of sound production. Singers spend a large portion of their time learning how to optimize breath support, so it is not surprising that any respiratory impairment can cause difficulties. For asthmatics, bronchospasms impair exhalation airflow, typically resulting in laryngeal hyperfunction. There are different severities of asthma, and in some cases mild or episodic cases can go undiagnosed. One such example is exercised-induced asthma, and the more specific form called airway reactivity induced asthma in singers (ARIAS) caused by airway drying during singing performance.[1] In singers/actors who also are required to dance, this additional exercise can impair their singing further.

Involvement of a pulmonologist, or lung specialist, is important for management. Pulmonary function tests help establish the diagnosis and monitor the treatment of this disease. If the asthma is allergy induced, including an allergist is helpful. Undiagnosed or under-treated laryngeal reflux can make asthma more symptomatic and harder to treat. It is important to inform your physician that you are a singer to avoid treatments that can be deleterious to your voice, and it will also help the pulmonologist understand the importance of optimizing your respiratory function and minimizing or avoiding the use of oral inhalers (especially those containing steroids).

References

1. Cohn, J.R., Sataloff, R.T., Spiegel, J.R., Fish, J.E., Kennedy, K. Airway reactivity-induced asthma in singers (ARIAS), *J Voice*. 1991; 5(4): 332–337.

29

Sing when you're sick

Deciding whether to sing while sick can be difficult. For example, a singer should not sing in a suboptimal state for a small, non-career defining performance; but one may gently push oneself to sing for a major audition. During your career, there will be times when you will be asked to perform injured. A director or conductor's ultimate goal is producing an outstanding event, and that does not necessarily take into account the health of, or risk to, a singer. In some cases, performing may be safe and warranted; but there will be times when withdrawing from a performance is more important in order avoid permanent injury to the singer's voice, and sometimes to the singer's reputation.

If a singer has an upper respiratory infection (viral or bacterial) without laryngitis, he or she might notice that the sound has changed because of nasal obstruction or pharyngeal swelling that affect self-perception (sometimes more than the perception of listeners). With lower respiratory infections, the power source may be impaired resulting in vocal strain. The sick singer should try to avoid throat clearing and coughing, as these activities may lead to vocal fold injury. Singing can be accomplished safely if the singer can sing "by feel" without changing technique in response to altered auditory feedback, but it should be done cautiously and with the guidance of a laryngologist.

If the singer has laryngitis in addition to the upper respiratory infection, he or she should be aware that there is potential for vocal fold edema and capillary fragility. These changes can increase the risk of vocal fold injury and hemorrhage. If a performance is not imminent, voice rest can minimize injury during the recovery process. If a singer has an imminent performance, he or she must weigh the pros and cons of performing. If he or she elects to perform, antibiotic therapy or steroids might improve vocal function, but they do not necessarily decrease injury risk. If the singer has taken blood thinners, such as over-the-counter cold medicines containing Aspirin, cancelation of performance should be considered seriously. Aspirin, or products containing aspirin, must be avoided to help prevent vocal fold hemorrhage. The decision whether to cancel should be made on a case-by-case basis with assistance of your voice team, including the laryngologist, SLP, SVS, singing teacher, manager, and others.

30

Don't drink enough water

Normal mucosal secretions are extremely important for free movement of the vibratory margin of the vocal folds. If vocal tract lubrication is suboptimal as a result of dehydration, or because of shifting the normal balance of serous and mucinous secretions, alterations in phonation occur. When singers develop this problem, thickening mucous results can be disastrous.

The performer who is sweating profusely due to being cloaked in heavy costumes or performing in a hot space should attend to replenishing fluids and minerals such as sodium, potassium, chloride, and magnesium. "Replenishment" should start at least several hours and ideally days in advance of the performance. The traveling performer may stay hydrated by extra water intake. The singer's body will tell him or her when hydration is adequate. When we are "dry" the kidneys tell the body to retain water, and urine becomes dark orange. When we are hydrated adequately, urine approaches the color of water. So, as the late Van Lawrence used to advise: Sing wet, pee pale. However, it also is important to recognize that some medications (including high doses of Vitamin C) can often alter urine color rendering coloration an invalid indicator of hydration. It is also possible to overdo water intake and cause electrolyte imbalance and serious medical problems.

Diuretics are potent medications that help the body eliminate excess fluid and should be taken only under a physician's supervision. An increase in circulating anti-diuretic hormone results in fluid retention in Reinke's space in the vocal folds, as well as other tissues. The fluid retained in the vocal fold during inflammation and hormonal shifts is protein bound, not free water. Diuretics do not remove this fluid effectively and can dehydrate the performer, resulting in decreased lubrication, thickened secretions, and persistently edematous vocal folds. Increased water intake can help compensate for this expected effect of a diuretic but also undermines the effectivness of the diuretic for treatment of conditions such as hypertension and Ménière's Disease.

31

Don't eat well

Preventative medicine is comprised of two elements: avoiding behaviors that are detrimental to health (smoking, excessive alcohol intake, drug use) and promoting behaviors that support good health (exercising, controlling stress, and eating a nutritious diet). Laryngeal and vocal health cannot be separated from general health and longevity. Nutritional status is extremely important. Inadequate nutrition invites illness and impairs optimal neuromuscular condition and performance by altering, or depriving the body of, the materials that make our bodies work.

There is more to nutrition than just maintaining good body weight. The foods we eat provide the chemical substrates necessary to build strength, improve and enhance body function, provide materials required by the immune system to fight infection, prevent inappropriate break down of body muscle, and for other essential functions. Improper dietary intake also can aggravate existing medical conditions, especially reflux. Consumption of appropriate foods and avoidance of acidic foods, onions, garlic, highly spiced foods, and other substances can decrease the symptoms of reflux.

Singers should remember that they are athletes. They require exercise to develop aerobic function and skeletal muscles. Like any other athlete, singers' bodies need the building blocks to make exercise effective. What we eat really does affect how we sing, and how long we sing.

32

Don't tell your doctors (allergists, pulmonologists, gastroenterologists, gynecologists, and others) that you're a singer

Diseases such as asthma, allergies, and reflux can affect the voice. Frequently, management of these illnesses requires involvement of physicians other than a singer's voice specialist (laryngologist/otolaryngologist). Examples (not inclusive) include allergists for asthma and allergy management; pulmonologists for asthma and other lung diseases; gastroenterologists for reflux disease, colon problems, and other maladies; endocrinologists for thyroid and sex hormone abnormalities; neurologists for tremor and other neurologic disorders; and rheumatologists for autoimmune diseases such as rheumatoid arthritis. Females need to inform their gynecologists/obstetricians that they are singers. Hormonal changes from menarche through menopause can affect the voice. Moreover, some medications used to treat hormonal imbalance and conditions such as endometriosis and postmenopause decrease in libido can result in untoward voice changes, some of which may be irreversible, especially changes caused by medications containing male hormones. Ideally, a singer should have a primary care doctor, who can help coordinate the singer's care.

Ideally, all doctors should understand the special considerations for maximizing a singer's health. Mismanagement of singers' medications is a frequent culprit in vocal problems. Uninformed physicians (and most of them are) may prescribe medication(s) that can be drying, cause inflammation and irritation of the larynx, or result in worse problems. It is the singer's responsibility to discuss his or her vocal requirements and any concerns regarding treatment with any treating physician. Concerns can be resolved by consultation with the singer's laryngologist.

33

Assume non-laryngeal surgery won't affect your voice

Typically, singers are aware of the risk of laryngeal surgery, but they are less familiar with the vocal risk associated with non-laryngeal surgery. Any procedure requiring general anesthesia usually requires the placement of an endotracheal tube (or breathing tube that passes between through the vocal folds). Even short-term intubations can lead to vocal fold injury and hoarseness. A singer undergoing a procedure should inform the anesthesiologist that he or she is a professional voice user, and the singer should request the most skilled member of the anesthesia team to perform the intubation using the smallest tube possible.

Surgeries involving the upper airway, such as the nasal cavity, oral cavity, and oropharynx, can affect resonance and articulation. Common examples of such procedures are tonsillectomies, septoplasty, and oropharyngeal surgery for sleep apnea. It may take several months for the voice to stabilize following the procedure, or in some cases scarring can affect the voice permanently. Frequently, an otolaryngologist performs these procedures and is more likely to be knowledgeable of the needs of voice patients. Despite this, the singer's concerns and voice use should be discussed with the surgeon prior to the procedure.

Surgeries that put the recurrent or superior laryngeal nerves at risk are also of concern to a singer. Such procedures include thoracic, cervical, thyroid, and intracranial procedures. The laryngeal nerves control motion of the vocal folds. If a singer needs one of these procedures, preoperative evaluation of the vocal folds' motion by a laryngologist will be helpful, especially later if an injury occurs or is suspected. Baseline information can be invaluable. Injury to the support musculature, such as abdominal or chest surgery, can impair breath support and phonation. Leg and foot surgery can impair a singer's ability to achieve and maintain proper stance and voice production. The singer should make the surgeon aware of his or her voice use and concerns prior to the procedure.

34

Assume laryngeal surgery will improve your voice

In general, a singer should be wary of a surgeon who is quick to operate on the larynx and vocal folds. There are exceptions, such as an airway obstruction or potentially malignant lesions that require prompt evaluation and treatment, but for the majority of patients, other treatment options should be considered prior to surgery. Voice therapy can be beneficial to the singer, in that it can improve technique, preventing further injury, and treat the underlying laryngeal abnormality. In some cases, voice therapy is all that is needed as the problem may resolve or the singer may learn to compensate safely.

If surgery is considered, all medical issues should be optimized prior to the procedure. This includes control of reflux. The risks of voice surgery can include (but are not limited to) scarring causing permanent hoarseness, recurrent vocal fold lesions, dental injury, and any airway compromise. Any singer electing to undergo voice surgery should discuss potential risks and complications with his or her surgeon prior to surgery. Even under ideal circumstances, scarring may persist or even worsen.

35

Assume your age (young and old) does not affect your voice

The larynx and vocal tract change throughout a singer's life. The first major milestone is puberty. The male's voice undergoes more drastic changes during puberty than the female's. The vocal tract and vocal folds lengthen, and the angle of the larynx becomes more pronounced. The fundamental frequency drops about an octave lower than a child's voice in males. The female voice changes during puberty are less pronounced, but there is still a slight drop in fundamental frequency. A singer may perform and practice during this time, but he or she (as well as the teacher) should take into account the dramatic events happening hormonally in the body during this time. The voice can be unstable, and it is difficult for a singer to control and predict the behavior of his or her fluctuating voice. Care should be taken to avoid overuse and injury during this time.

With aging, there is atrophy wasting of the laryngeal and thoracic muscles and arthrosis (stiffening, essentially) of the laryngeal joints. In women, menopause results in a decrease in progesterone and estrogen levels. The hormonal changes in women can cause dramatic changes affecting their singing voice. Singers may notice breathiness, hoarseness, and loss of vocal intensity, projection, range, and stamina with aging, among other problems. There are several options to help minimize these changes or restore the voice. These include voice therapy, hormone replacement therapy in women, and laryngeal medialization surgery (bringing the vocal folds closer together). Depending on the degree of impairment, your physician and voice team can help you decided the best treatment option.

36

Don't follow your doctor's advice

Caring for a singer's voice requires not only a knowledgeable physician, but also a cooperative patient. Frequently, correcting voice-related problems takes time as voice changes are progressive, often occurring over many years. Thus laryngologists may prescribe treatments that require considerable time commitments and social and work restrictions to achieve rehabilitation of the impaired voice.

Voice rest is a controversial topic among voice specialists. There is no clear consensus in the literature as to optimal duration of voice rest. It is commonly agreed that voice rest should be used for acute vocal fold injury, such as tears and hemorrhages, and in the postoperative period for patients undergoing voice surgery. Common sense would indicate that limiting phonation allows time for the vocal fold to heal and helps prevent further injury, but voice rest can cause social and financial hardship. The optimal duration of voice rest is not defined scientifically. Patients must rely on their physician's expertise and clinical experience to recommend the optimal duration of voice rest. Not following your doctor's advice can result in further damage and possibly permanent injury to the vocal folds.

Voice therapy should be viewed as a treatment tool but also an important part of voice maintenance. Frequently, early sessions are frustrating for the singer as the voice may worsen prior to improving and learning new techniques and methods can be difficult. Persistence and diligent work with the voice team is usually rewarded with an improved voice and easier phonation. Failure to comply with voice therapy can result in further damage and injury to the larynx.

37

Don't treat underlying
health issues

Numerous systemic illnesses can affect the voice. A few of the most common or troublesome are discussed in this chapter, including neurologic diseases, endocrine disorders, and autoimmune disease.

Essential tremor is the most common movement disorder and is likely under reported. Singers with this disorder may present with vocal tremor along with other bodily tremors. Treatments are not universally effective, but there are several options including anti-tremor medication, voice therapy, Botox injections, and deep brain stimulation. Parkinson's disease is associated commonly with hypo-adduction, or impaired vocal fold closure, resulting in a decrease in volume and breathiness. Voice tremor is frequently one of the early signs of the disease, and it can be treated with specialized voice therapy and medicines for Parkinson's disease. As the disease progresses, surgery may be needed to improve glottic closure, that is bring the vocal folds closer together to increase loudness and decrease vocal effect.

The body is regulated by a complex set of hormones produced by endocrine glands such as the thyroid and adrenal glands. Hypo- and hyperthyroidism, or low or high levels of thyroid hormones, respectively, are two of the more common endocrine causes of vocal complaints. Hyperthyroidism can increase stimulation of the laryngeal muscles and may cause tremor and hoarseness in addition to generalized anxiety. Common symptoms of hypothyroidism include swelling of the vocal folds, voice weakness, a generalized fatigue and vocal muffling described commonly as "a veil over the voice." Testing for thyroid function in vocal disorders is important to rule out an easily treatable cause of a voice disorders.

Autoimmune diseases are disorders in which an individual's own cells cause inflammation and attack parts of one's own body. Some of these diseases that affect the larynx are myasthenia gravis, rheumatoid arthritis, lupus, thyroiditis, and granulomatosis with polyangiitis. For example, rheumatoid arthritis can cause stiffness and inflammation of the laryngeal joints restricting the movement of the vocal folds, and potentially can cause shortness of breath and hoarseness. Commonly, autoimmune disease requires treatment with steroids and immune-suppressing (mild chemotherapy) drugs to decrease the inflammation and tissue injury.

Many systemic diseases can affect the larynx, some of which (like reflux) are discussed in other chapters. Early diagnosis and treatment are important to maintain the vocal health of a singer. Having a diligent primary care doctor, medical specialists, and a voice specialist working together help insure prompt diagnosis and treatment.

38

Don't take care of your mental health

The relationship between a singer's mental health and vocal health is complex. Mental health issues can have a negative effect on both speaking and singing and vice versa.

Neglecting your mental health can affect the voice in varying ways. Psychological disorders may impair a singer's ability to sleep and may cause the singer to develop substance abuse problems, which were discussed in more detail in other chapters. Depression and bipolar disorders may alter the singer's motivation and drive and diminish his or her focus, thus affecting the voice itself, as well as artistic expression in performance. Anxiety disorders may affect the singer's ability to perform or interact with other professionals. In some cases, psychological disorders precede the development of voice disorders, but primary vocal problems can be very troublesome to a singer and often give rise to anxiety and depression.

Involvement of a trained medical specialist is important for proper diagnosis and treatment. In some people an underlying medical condition, such as an endocrine abnormality, can cause psychiatric symptoms. Screening for these possible conditions is important. For some, psychological therapy can be very beneficial, while others may need medication in addition to therapy. It is important to tell your mental health specialist that you are a singer, as some psychiatric medications can have negative effects on the voice. For example, lithium used to treat bipolar disorders can cause increased urination producing dehydration, which can cause drying of the mucosa. It is important to discuss the side effects and their negative impact on your voice. Your mental health care provider can work with you and your laryngologist to find the optimal combination of medications.

Stress can aggravate underlying psychological disease, and stress alone can affect the mental health of a singer. Singers may suffer the symptoms of acute stress, such as heart racing and increased or decreased salivation, and with chronic stress they may develop chronic fatigue, lack of motivation, pain syndromes, and multiple somatic complaints. The first step in management of stress is identifying its presence. Once the singer has identified the stressors, he or she may be able to eliminate them or mitigate their effects on the voice and mental health.

39

Ignore your eating disorder

Eating disorders are now epidemic and recognized worldwide. Singers and others in the entertainment business with its requisite media exposure, including dancers and professional models, are especially vulnerable to these debilitating "secret" illnesses. No one can approach full vocal potential while chained to an eating disorder.

The young singer may not consider disordered eating abnormal but rather a necessary part of striving for perfection in service of his/her art. Sometimes singers who fear that their technical proficiency is not equal to that of their classmates will adopt an attitude that if they cannot be the best in the class they can be the thinnest. Weight control by restricting food intake can induce more difficulties.

Bulimia nervosa and anorexia nervosa both involve disordered eating. Anorexia is a mental disorder that involves aversion to food and great fear of becoming obese, associated with a disturbed body image. It affects young women most commonly and can be life-threatening. Bulimia involves episodes of rapid consumption of large quantities of food in short periods of time, followed by purging using laxatives, diuretics, or self-induced vomiting. It also may be accompanied by vigorous exercise and fasting. Associated feelings of guilt are common, as is depression. It may occur sporadically or be a chronic problem.

Bulimia and binge eating may be more prevalent than commonly realized. They have been estimated to occur in as many as 1.5–3.5% of females, particularly adolescents and young adults, including vocalists and dancers. Males also are affected, although at lower rates. Bulimia also may be associated with anorexia nervosa.

Vomiting in bulimia produces signs and symptoms similar to those caused by severe, chronic reflux, as well as thinning of tooth enamel. In addition to posterior laryngitis and pharyngitis, laryngeal findings associated with bulimia include sub-epithelial vocal fold hemorrhages, superficial telangiectasia (prominent, abnormal blood vessels) of the vocal fold mucosa, and vocal fold scarring. Clinicians must be attentive to the potential for anorexia, bulimia, and exercise addiction in the maintenance of a desirable body appearance in performers.

There is enormous popular interest in the use of appetite suppressants in weight management. Many myths persist about proper weight management approaches in singers and the value and/or risk of weight loss. The availability and popularity of appetite suppressant drugs, and mass marketing approaches that made them available in franchised weight loss centers, led many Americans to explore their use in the 1990s. These medications had limited efficacy in changing metabolism and craving, and many patients took these drugs in combinations that were never approved for concomitant use. The drugs were withdrawn from the market voluntarily by their manufacturers in 1997 due to significant risks of cardiac (heart) valve damage and pulmonary (lung) hypertension.

40

Deny that you have a voice problem

"Hoarseness" is an annoyance that many people tend to ignore, but any persistent abnormal change in the voice – including a breathy, raspy, or strained quality – should be evaluated. A little hoarseness can be the sign of a big problem. If ignored, the problem can get worse. Voice problems can limit productivity in the workplace and damage quality of life.

Hoarseness can have many different causes, including a cold, allergy, or gastroesophageal reflux; but hoarseness that lasts for more than three weeks can be a sign of serious problems, including cancer.

Cancers can occur in anyone, including young singers who do not smoke. Singers work hard to entertain the public. They spend numerous hours training and performing. However, musical prowess can lead to stress and a tragic fall from grace caused by addictions, mental issues, and in some cases physical injuries that lead to problems such as vocal fold nodules. There is a veritable conspiracy of silence around the occurrence of nodes, polyps, and other problems that plague even the greatest opera singers. It can feel like heresy to talk about vocal problems. A performer may deny that there is an issue because it might affect his or her ability to be hired; but more serious psychological problems may be responsible for the denial[1]. Whatever the cause, both the voice change and the reason for denial should be evaluated and treated promptly.

References

1. Rosen, D.C. and Sataloff, R.T. *Psychology of Voice Disorders*. San Diego, CA: Singular Publishing Group, Inc.; 1997.

41

Clear your throat

Chronic throat clearing can be a particularly harmful behavior. The forceful and excessive closure of the vocal folds can lead to vocal fold trauma causing vocal fold hemorrhages, tears and masses, which can be detrimental to a singer's career.

The urge to clear your throat can come from chronic problems such as laryngopharyngeal reflux (LPR) and allergies, or from acute issues such as upper respiratory infections (i.e. the common cold), which are discussed in other chapters. In some cases, it may be due to other noxious stimuli (e.g. cigarette smoke, perfumes, chemical cleaners, and others) or secondary to abnormal laryngeal sensation. If the etiology is noxious stimuli, avoidance is recommended, and in the case of abnormal laryngeal irritation from a condition such as LPR, medications and life style changes may be prescribed.

A voice team, and in particular a laryngologist, can be helpful in the diagnosis and treatment of the underlying problem. Occasionally, a diagnosis is not made, but the voice team consisting of a speech-language pathologist and singing-voice specialist can aid in utilizing techniques to avoid potentially traumatic throat clearing. Frequently, the singer is advised to swallow when he or she feels the need to clear his or her throat, and to increase hydration to help with dryness and thick mucus. Eliminating this harmful behavior is very beneficial to singers.

42

Don't treat dental/oral cavity disease

Any oral cavity problem, from painful sores to poor deteriation to dental fracture, can affect singing in performers of any age, as can temporomandibular joint (TMJ) problems. These conditions will not be discussed in detail but should not be ignored. However, oral cavity changes associated with aging are very common and may be particularly troublesome to singers. So we will address them in greater detail. Loss of dentition may alter occlusion and articulation, causing disturbing problems, especially for professional voice users and wind instrumentalists. These difficulties may be avoided to some extent by having impressions made while dentition is still normal (when we're young). Dentures that are more similar to the person's natural teeth can then be fashioned and will be easier for the performer to use without unconscious, compensatory changes in the vocal mechanism.

Although salivary glands lose up to about 30% of their parenchymal tissue over a lifetime, salivary secretion remains adequate in most healthy, non-medicated people throughout life. However, changes in the oral mucosa are similar to those occurring in the skin (thinning and dehydration). They render oral mucosa in the elderly more susceptible to injury, and the sensation of dry mouth maybe especially disturbing to singers. Oral cancers also comprise about 5% of all malignancies, and 95% of oral cancers occur in people over 40 years of age. Cancers in the head and neck may result in profound voice dysfunction.

Halitosis maybe a sign of anunderlying medical conditions, such as laryngopharyngeal reflux or acute sinusitis, that warrants proper medical diagnosis and treatment. It is useful for singers and their health care providers to recognize the social and medical importance of halitosis, to admit its presence, to investigate it systematically, and to eliminate it whenever possible. Oral hygiene problems are a common cause of halitosis and are usually easy to identify and cure. Food or epithelial debris may be trapped between teeth, in areas of periodontal disease, on the dorsal tongue surface, or in mucosal pockets and creases of the tonsils (cryptic tonsils). Dental appliances such as dentures and bridges also frequently permit collection of such debris, which is broken down by anaerobic and gram-negative bacteria. "Coated tongue" similarly causes bad breath by the breakdown of debris by bacteria creating bad breath. Chronic periodontal disease or gingivitis with bleeding from the gums produces a particularly unattractive odor that can be detected following oral bleeding from other causes such as trauma, bleeding disorders, tumors, and hemorrhage from the pharynx or tonsils. Any oral condition that impairs hydration also predisposes to halitosis of oral origin. Such conditions include dehydration from insufficient fluid intake commonly seen in the elderly, chronic mouth breathing, medications such as anti-histamines and diuretics, collagen vascular disease, Sjogren's syndrome, and radiation therapy among others. In most cases, adequate hydration, excellent oral hygiene including brushing the tongue as well as brushing and flossing the teeth, and routine dental and periodontal care can suppress odors of oral origin. If halitosis is untreated, word gets out; and singers may lose invitations to perform with other singers even if their voices are still good.

Dental disease, especially temporomandibular joint dysfunction, introduces muscle tension in the head and neck, which is transmitted to the larynx directly through the muscular attachments between the mandible and hyoid (tongue) bone and indirectly as generalized increased muscle tension. These problems often result in decreased vocal range, vocal fatigue, and change in the quality or placement of a voice. Such tension often is accompanied by excess muscle activity, especially pulling of the tongue posteriorly. This hyperfunctional behavior acts through hyoid attachments to disrupt the balance between the intrinsic and laryngeal musculature. The history in such patients should always include information about other musical activities, including instruments other than the voice, especially single reed instruments.

43

Don't protect your larynx from injury

Injury to the front of the larynx itself can be devastating. Usually, such injuries result from motor vehicle accidents in which the neck strikes the steering wheel or during altercations. However, there are many other common causes of laryngeal injury. Elbow injuries to the larynx occur commonly to people playing basketball, ice hockey, and other sports. We have seen patients with laryngeal fractures that occurred on stage when one singer was struck in the neck accidentally by the arms-spread-wide gesture of an enthusiastic fellow performer.

Direct trauma to the larynx can produce hemorrhage into the vocal folds, dislocation of the arytenoid cartilages, injury to the cricothyroid joint (which is needed to allow normal changes in pitch) and fracture of other laryngeal cartilages. Such injuries have the life-threatening potential of airway obstruction. They can be avoided in many cases by proper use of seatbelts with shoulder restraints. Singers should avoid (or be very careful playing) sports in which the risk of being hit in the neck is high. They should also be careful about "grand gestures" from other performers on stage; and if flailing arm movements are required artistically, stage blocking should be designed to help minimize the risk of accidental strikes to the front of the neck. However, when anterior neck trauma occurs, immediate visualization of the larynx by a skilled laryngologist is essential. Laryngeal injuries are frequently worse than they appear to be at first. They need to be evaluated expertly to determine the nature of injury not only to the laryngeal cartilages (which ossify, becoming bone-like as we age), but also to the soft tissues of the larynx, including the vocal folds, and to the nerves, which can also be damaged by traumatic injury. The best chance for full recovery from the effects of laryngeal trauma comes with prompt diagnosis and treatment.

44

Don't realize that various bodily injuries outside the vocal tract may affect the voice

Various bodily injuries outside the vocal tract may have profound effects on the voice. Whiplash, for example, commonly causes changes in technique, with consequent voice fatigue, loss of range, difficulty singing softly, and other problems. These problems derive from the neck muscle spasm, abnormal neck posture secondary to pain, and consequent hyperfunctional voice use. Lumbar, abdominal, head, chest, supraglottic, and extremity injuries also may affect vocal technique and be responsible for dysphonia that prompts the voice patient to seek medical attention.[1]

Serious injuries to the head producing unconsciousness may be fatal. Even when people recover from skull fractures or closed head injury, subtle brain dysfunction may persist for many months or even permanently[1]. This usually includes slight personality change, emotional lability, impaired memory, sometimes difficulty reading or speaking, and often nonspecific loss of "sharpness." Such impairments may be serious impediments to healthy singing. Head trauma also may be associated with hearing loss, which is most likely to occur if there is a blow directly to the ear or one severe enough to cause unconsciousness. If hearing loss is found, counseling and rehabilitation usually avert vocal problems. However, if hearing loss goes unrecognized, the singer may "oversing" to compensate for the hearing impairment. Similar problems occur in actors or other professional speakers.[2]

Injury to the nose, such as a nasal fracture, can produce nasal obstruction. This alters the production of certain sounds and may force the singer to breathe unfiltered, unhumidified cold air through his or her mouth. This may result in voice irritation, especially in dusty or dry environments. Injury to the oral cavity, including surgical injury during tonsillectomy, changes a singer's sound. The shape and pliability of the tongue, palate, and pharyngeal muscles are important. Although voice alterations caused by minor swelling or scarring in these areas are often more obvious to the singer or actor than they are to listeners, they are hazardous because performers tend to try to compensate for them. Many singers develop hyperfunctional technique in attempts to overcome them.[2]

Chest and abdominal injuries may occur through motor vehicle accidents, surgery, or other trauma. Usually, they result in temporary muscle dysfunction. Some injuries leave residual problems. If all or part of one lung is lost, voice technique may need to be modified. Similar problems may occur if lung function is impaired by inhalation injury. One of the conditions of greatest risk for voice abuse is when a singer is nearly out of breath. Singers with lung impairment must be careful to alter their phrasing to permit extra breaths, rather than attempting to sing extended phrases as they had prior to the injury. In addition, a vigorous program of medically supervised aerobic rehabilitation is advised. Following abdominal injuries, weaknesses in the abdominal muscle wall, such as ventral hernias, may persist. These may interfere with the support mechanism and require surgical repair.[2]

Back muscles are integral to voice support. Thoracic, lumbar, and sacral injury can interfere with voice performance. Such injuries may cause nerve dysfunction and consequent weakness in muscles used for respiration and support. Thoracic back pain may limit inspiration, and lumbosacral back pain may impede firm contraction of the abdominal and back muscles for support. This may alter the balance of muscle function which is essential for efficient phonation. These problems result commonly in unconscious attempts at compensation that often lead to hyperfunctional technique. This not only is counterproductive in terms of quality and endurance, but also may lead to structural injuries of the vocal folds.

References

1. Mandel, S., Sataloff, R.T. and Schapiro, S. *Minor Head Trauma: Assessment, Management, and Rehabilitation.* New York, NY: Springer-Verlag; 1993.

2. Sataloff, R.T. *Professional Voice: The Science and Art of Clinical Care,* Third Edition. San Diego, CA: Plural Publishing, Inc.; 2005.

45

Expose yourself to environmental irritants

Exposure to environmental irritants is a well-recognized cause of voice dysfunction. Smoke, dehydration, pollution, and allergens may produce hoarseness, frequent throat clearing, and voice fatigue. These problems sometimes can be improved by environmental modification, medication, or simply breathing through the nose rather than the mouth, as the nose humidifies and filters incoming air.

Performing outside brings its own hazards, such as insect bites and precipitous changes in the weather, including wind, humidity, extreme heat or cold, rain, and lightning. Substances used for special effects, materials used in scene building, and makeup constitute possible hazards and toxicities for the performer. Costumes, wigs, various makeups, even the paint used on sets can be a source of toxic exposure, irritation, and allergies. Special effects such as fogs can be unpleasant as well as risky for those performers, especially singers, who may have underlying respiratory ailments.[1]

Any mucosal irritant can disrupt the delicate vocal mechanism. Allergies to dust and mold are aggravated commonly during rehearsals and performances, especially in older theaters and concert halls, because of numerous curtains, backstage trappings, and dressing facilities that are rarely cleaned thoroughly. The drying effects of cold air and dry heat also may affect mucosal secretions, leading to decreased lubrication, scratchy voice, and tickling cough. Environmental pollution is responsible for the presence of toxic substances and conditions encountered daily. Inhalation of toxic pollutants may affect the voice adversely by direct laryngeal injury, by causing pulmonary dysfunction that results in voice maladies, or through impairments elsewhere in the vocal tract. Ingested substances, especially those that have neurolaryngologic (voice nerves) effects, may also adversely affect voice.

A history of recent travel suggests other sources of mucosal irritation. The air in airplanes is extremely dry and airplanes are noisy. Environmental changes also can be disruptive. A history of recent travel should also suggest jetlag and generalized fatigue, which may be potent detriments to good vocal function.

References

1. US Dep of Health and Human Services, Public Health Service, National Toxicology Program (NTP). Report on Carcinogens. 10th ed. Research Triangle Park, NC: NTP; 2002.

46

Don't realize that hearing loss can affect the voice

Hearing impairment can cause vocal strain, particularly if the person has sensorineural (nerve) hearing loss and is unaware of it. This condition may lead people to speak or sing more loudly than they realize. Singers and other musicians depend on good hearing to match pitch, monitor vocal or sound quality, and provide feedback and direction for adjustments during performance. The importance of good hearing among performing artists has been underappreciated. Although well-trained musicians are usually careful to protect their voices or hands, they may subject their ears to unnecessary damage and thereby threaten their musical careers. Hearing is a critical part of a musician's instrument. Consequently, it is important for him/her to understand how the ear works, how to take care of it, what can go wrong with it, and how to avoid hearing loss from preventable injury.

Various methods have been devised to help protect the hearing of performers. For example, many singers and other musicians wear ear protectors. They may not feel comfortable wearing ear protection during a performance, but may take cautionary measures during practice. Singers and instrumentalists need to be made more aware of the hazards of noise exposure and find ways to avoid or reduce its effects whenever possible. Because many singers and instrumentalists practice or perform 4 to 8 hours a day (sometimes more), noise exposure levels may be significant. Although noise induced hearing loss usually is symmetric, asymmetric hearing loss is a common finding in classical musicians and especially among violinists. Ear protection devices have changed tremendously over the years, and there are more sophisticated and suitable models available now that cater to musicians. The importance of using new, more appropriate ear protectors for professional musicians should be stressed especially because the relationship between music exposure and noise induced hearing loss has become clear. Singers need to be made more aware of the hazards of noise exposure and find ways to avoid or reduce its effects. They also should be careful to avoid exposure to potentially damaging avocational noise, such as loud music through headphones, chainsaws, snowmobiles, gunfire, motorcycles, and power tools. Singers depend on their hearing almost as much as they do on their voices. It is important not to take such a valuable and delicate structure as the ear for granted. Like voice, the ear must be understood and protected if the singer or other musician is to enjoy a long, happy, and successful career.

47

Sing or play in the wrong environment or with the wrong equipment

When, where, how, and what instrumentalists play can affect the potential for music-related injuries; many singers also are instrumentalists but do not recognize that playing instruments may affect health that impacts singing. The following list of factors influencing the musical environment include the number, duration, length, and intensity of rehearsals; degree of difficulty of the repertoire and the musicians' familiarity with it; legibility of the score; lighting conditions allowing for the reading of music; acoustic properties of the environment; the musicians proximity to certain other instruments; the ambient temperature affecting both the instrument and the voice; and the comfort and proper positioning of the seating.

For substances such as some used for special effects, materials used in scene building, and makeup, material data sheets are available that specify the chemical constituents and their hazards and possible toxicities, as well as proper handling. Costumes, wigs, various makeups, even the paint used on the sets can be sources of toxic exposure, irritation, and allergies. Special effects such as fogs can be unpleasant as well as risky, especially for those with underlying respiratory ailments.

All need to be considered as possible offending agents when an actor or singer presents with an unknown respiratory problem or rash.

The importance of using ear protectors for instrumentalists should be stressed, especially because the relationship between even orchestral music exposure and noise induced hearing loss has been established. Problems exist in classical orchestras, not just rock bands. Many singers and other musicians, especially in rock bands, wear ear protectors. Singers and musicians often need to be aware of the hazards of noise exposure and find ways to avoid or reduce its effects whenever possible. When a singer's hearing is impaired, vocal performance may be impaired.

Another very important and under-considered piece of equipment for singers is the chair. Seat modification is only a battle in the war against back discomfort. Singers, along with other seated workers and students, are often unintentional victims of poorly designed seating. Back pain in a sitting position has several causes: poorly designed chairs, deconditioned backs, inadequate back awareness, and inability to maintain an erect posture with little muscular effort because of chair design. These problems can undermine support and lead to hoarseness and voice fatigue during choir rehearsals, for example.

It is extremely helpful to assess the room or hall prior to a singing engagement. The singer should investigate acoustics, type of microphones and speakers available, room temperature, availability of water, lighting on the stage, tuning adequacy of the piano, and presence or absence of a stage manager, among other factors. This allows for connections to be made in advance (or at least recognized), decreasing stress during the performance.

48

Play a wind instrument (especially, badly)

Wind instrument players may develop pharyngoceles or laryngoceles that present as a large airbag in the neck, which stand out as they play. They sometimes interfere with performance and require treatment. The most common complaints reported by wind instrumentalists are fatigue during playing, lip and throat pain, loss of upper range, and loss of ability to sustain long notes. Expression of a musical composition of a woodwind and brass melody requires precise neuromuscular control of the orofacial complex. The mouth and associated musculature are the crucial apparatus for the wind instrument and instrumentalists. For some musicians, the musical melody becomes a medical malady through trauma, misuse, or overuse of the orofacial structures. Overuse syndrome is characterized by pain and tenderness in the lips, tongue, muscles, and joints as a consequence of excessive use, manifesting itself as loss of agility and accuracy. All of these problems acquired through playing may affect singing as well. The individual variability of the orofacial structures and their adaptability throughout life should be considered when a musician initially chooses a wind instrument.

The ease of positioning the instrument relative to the anterior teeth contributes to forming the embouchure, and some dental and facial patterns facilitate the adaptation of the mouth to the mouthpiece. Ignoring the physical requirements can result in the selection of an instrument that is not suited to the musician's morphology, which may limit his or her ability to play to full potential. Moreover, the mismatch may lead to temporomandibular joint (TMJ) pain and neck and facial muscle tension that impair singing. Poor control, muscle fatigue, sores on the lips, or pain of the temporomandibular joints can all compromise the embouchure. When playing a wind instrument, the tone and pitch are varied by alteration of the size of the lip aperture, change in the tension of the embouchure musculature, and thus changes in lip pressure. Changes in head position, which result in compensatory changes in mandibular position and changes in the pharyngeal airway, also alter tonal quality.[1]

Dental and skeletal changes in wind instrumentalists have been noted in the literature. Such differences include the inclination of the maxillary and mandibular incisors (giant teeth), slight increase in labial inclination (leaning toward the lips) of both maxillary and mandibular incisors, tendency for the mandibular (lower jaw) dental arch to be decreased in width with an increase in length attributed to the sustained contraction of the muscles at the corner of the mouth when playing wind instruments. Pang[2] concluded that for the growing individual, the effect of playing a wind instrument on the position of the anterior teeth is unpredictable and that only on a group basis can a class of wind instruments be theorized to alter skeletal and dental relationships. Cheney[3] noted that maxillary dental protrusion was considered a problem by all of the brass players whom he had classified as having forward tooth position. The gentle protrusion was reported to interfere with slipped placement and required greater forward posturing of the lower jaw to form the embouchure. Anterior dental over-bites were a problem for brass players but were particularly disturbing to woodwind musicians, because they experienced difficulty in preventing the escape of air from the corners of the mouth during prolonged playing.

Vocalists often extend the jaw beyond the normal range of motion, and the relationship between the airway, jaw position, and the prolonged mouth opening associated with singing may aggravate the underlying

TMJ condition.[4] Painful catching or locking of the TMJ in a wide opened mouth position interferes with singing and is often associated with temporal headaches. Singing requires precise positioning of the mandible, backward tongue pull, and tongue compression, all of which can influence the facial skeleton. All can also be affected by playing wind instruments.

As in similar performance problems of singers, some wind instrumentalists develop performance dysfunctions due to pulmonary dysfunction, particularly unrecognized asthma. Performance using the woodwind or brass musical instruments requires consistent control over the stream of expired air. This is true for singers, in whom pulmonary and vocal fold level aerodynamics have been studied more extensively.[1]

In addition to all of the problems noted above, playing wind instruments also involves use of the larynx itself. Vocal folds open and close in many instrumentalists when they play rapid runs and often at other times. Part of expert wind playing involves relaxation of the muscles of the throat and larynx, and sophistication of laryngeal articulation. These are also goals of vocal training. If an instrumentalist is an expert wind player well-suited to his/her instrument, it should be possible to play a wind instrument without affecting singing adversely. However, if the instrumentalist is not an expert, tensions and injuries of the vocal tract acquired while playing a wind instrument can damage the ability to sing.

References

1. Sataloff RT, Brandfonbrener AG, Lederman RJ, (editors). Performing Arts Medicine, 3rd edition. 2010 Science and Medicine, Inc.

2. Pang A. Relation of musical wind instruments to malocclusion. J Am Dent Assoc 1976, 92: 565–570.

3. Cheney EA. Adaption to embouchure as a function of dentofacial complex. Am J Orthod. 1949; 35: 440–456.

4. Amorino S, Taddy J. Temporomandibular joint disorders and the singing voice. NATS J. 1994; 50(1): 3–14.

49

Don't get second opinions

Visits to a doctor can be expensive. Many singers hesitate to go in the first place. Too many decide not to spend the money to get a second opinion, even when they are not confident in the opinion they have received from the first doctor.

Voice care is an art. It is also a relatively new medical science, as mentioned elsewhere in this book. There are few ear, nose, and throat doctors with specialty training in care of the professional voice. In fact, there are fewer trained laryngologists than there are otolaryngology training programs. Consequently, even today, many excellent ear, nose, and throat doctors do not have expertise in the management of voice problems, and especially in the complex issues that must be considered in diagnosing and treating singers.

Unless a singer is absolutely certain that he/she is in the hands of someone who is truly expert in caring for voice disorders, seeking a second opinion from a physician who sub-specializes in voice care often is wise. This is true especially when the first physician has found no cause for the singer's problem ("there's nothing wrong with your vocal folds") without providing helpful insight, or when surgery has been recommended without clear, compelling, and sensible reasons that the singer understands.

Second opinions may be costly, but they are less costly than the avoidable end of a singing career. However, it is essential that the "second opinion" be truly expert. Getting the opinion of two otherwise excellent ear, nose, and throat doctors, neither of whom know anything about professional voice care, is not sufficient.

50

Don't follow the suggestions in this book

These guidelines are designed to help singers optimize and perfect the natural talent provided to them and to avoid abuse/misuse that may lead to inferior performance and to vocal injury. The human's ability to produce beautiful sound with his or her voice is amazing. Small variations in this process can cause immense changes in the overall sound produced. Singers must be aware of potential pitfalls and ways to avoid them. Some of these hazards may not be critically detrimental initially, but over time they may cause serious damage to the voice. Following the rules outlined in this text will provide singers with the foundation necessary to have a lasting, healthy singing career.

Suggested Readings

The following is a suggested readings list of selected other books by the Authors

Sataloff, R.T. *Professional Voice: The Science and Art of Clinical Care*, Third Edition. San Diego, CA: Plural Publishing, Inc.; 2005.

Sataloff, R.T. (Ed.). *Vocal Health and Pedagogy*, Second Edition. San Diego, CA: Plural Publishing, Inc.; 2006.

Rubin, J., Sataloff, R.T. and Korovin, G. *Diagnosis and Treatment of Voice Disorders*, Fourth Edition. San Diego, CA: Plural Publishing, Inc. 2014

Rosen, D.C. and Sataloff, R.T. *Psychology of Voice Disorders*. San Diego, CA: Singular Publishing Group, Inc.; 1997.

Sataloff, R.T., Katz, P.O., Sataloff, D.M. and Hawkshaw, M.J. *Reflux Laryngitis and Related Disorders*, Fourth Edition. San Diego, CA: Plural Publishing, Inc.; 2013.

Sataloff, R.T., Brandfonbrener, A. and Lederman, R. (Eds.). *Performing Arts Medicine*, Third Edition. Narberth, PA: Science and Medicine; 2010.

Sataloff, R.T., Hawkshaw, M.J., Sataloff, J.B., DeFatta, R.A., and Eller, R.L. Atlas of Laryngoscopy, Third Edition. San Diego, California: Plural Publishing, Inc.; 2012.

Sataloff, R.T. and Sataloff, J. *Occupational Hearing Loss*, Third Edition. New York, NY: Taylor & Francis, Inc.; 2006.

Smith, B. and Sataloff, R.T. *Choral Pedagogy*, Third Edition. San Diego, CA: Plural Publishing, Inc.; 2013.

Smith, B. and Sataloff, R.T. *Choral Pedagogy and the Older Singer*. San Diego, CA: Plural Publishing, Inc.; 2012.

Sataloff, R.T. *Medical Musings*. Oxford: Compton Publishing Ltd.; 2014.

Author Biographies

Robert T. Sataloff, M.D., D.M.A., F.A.C.S. is Professor and Chairman, Department of Otolaryngology-Head and Neck Surgery and Senior Associate Dean for Clinical Academic Specialties, Drexel University College of Medicine. He is also Adjunct Professor in the departments of Otolaryngology – Head and Neck Surgery at Thomas Jefferson University and the University of Pennsylvania, as well as Temple University; and 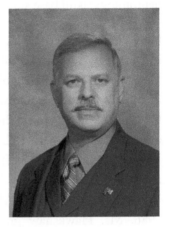 on the faculty of the Academy of Vocal Arts. Dr. Sataloff is also a professional singer and singing teacher, and he served as Conductor of the Thomas Jefferson University Choir over a period of nearly four decades. He holds an undergraduate degree from Haverford College in Music Theory and Composition, graduated from Jefferson Medical College, Thomas Jefferson University, received a Doctor of Musical Arts in Voice Performance from Combs College of Music; and he completed his Residency in Otolaryngology - Head and Neck Surgery and a Fellowship in Otology, Neurotology and Skull Base Surgery at the University of Michigan. Dr. Sataloff is Chairman of the Boards of Directors of the Voice Foundation and of the American Institute for Voice and Ear Research. He has also served as Chairman of the Board of Governors of Graduate Hospital; President of the American Laryngological Association, the International Association of Phonosurgery, and the Pennsylvania Academy of Otolaryngology – Head and Neck Surgery; and in numerous other leadership positions. Dr. Sataloff is Editor-in-Chief of the *Journal of Voice*, Editor-in-Chief of *Ear, Nose and Throat Journal*, Editor-in-Chief of the *Journal of Case Reports in Medicine*, Associate Editor of the *Journal of Singing*, and on the editorial boards of numerous otolaryngology journals. He has written over 1,000 publications, including 50 books. His medical practice is limited to care of the professional voice and to otology/neurotology/skull base surgery.

Mary J. Hawkshaw, B.S.N., R.N., CORLN is Research Associate Professor in the Department of Otolaryngology – Head and Neck Surgery at Drexel University College of Medicine. She has been associated with Dr. Robert Sataloff, Philadelphia Ear, Nose & Throat Associates and the American Institute for Voice & Ear Research (AIVER) since 1986. Ms. Hawkshaw graduated from Shadyside Hospital School of Nursing in Pittsburgh, Pennsylvania and 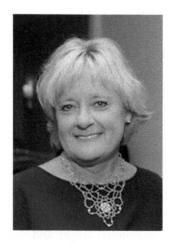 received a Bachelor of Science degree in Nursing from Thomas Jefferson University in Philadelphia. In addition to her specialized clinical activities, she has been involved extensively in research and teaching. She mentors medical students, residents, and laryngology fellows, and has been involved in teaching research, writing and editing for nearly three decades. In collaboration with Dr. Sataloff, she has co-authored more than 170 articles, 70 book chapters, and 10 textbooks. A member of the Editorial Boards of the *Journal of Voice* and *Ear, Nose and Throat Journal*, she has served as Secretary/Treasurer of AIVER since 1988 and was named Executive Director

January 2000. She has served on the Board of Directors of the Voice Foundation since 1990. Ms. Hawkshaw has been an active member of the Society of Otorhinolaryngology and Head-Neck Nurses since 1998. She is recognized nationally and internationally for her extensive contributions to care of the professional voice.

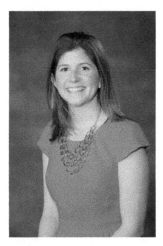

Jaime Eaglin Moore, M.D. is an otolaryngologist and laryngologist. Dr. Moore is board certified by the American Board of Otolaryngology. Dr. Moore received her Doctor of Medicine degree from Eastern Virginia Medical School, and she completed a residency in Otolaryngology – Head and Neck Surgery at Virginia Commonwealth University in Richmond, Virginia. She was a fellow in laryngology and care of the professional voice at the American Institute for Voice and Ear Research. Author of numerous publications and a Fellow Editor for the *Journal of Voice*, Dr. Moore is an assistant professor at Virginia Commonwealth University Health System.

Amy L. Rutt, D.O. is an Instructor in the Department of Otolaryngology-Head and Neck Surgery at Drexel University College of Medicine in Philadelphia, Pennsylvania. Dr Rutt attended King's College, where she graduated with a Bachelor of Science and Physician's Assistant degree. She received her medical degree from the Philadelphia College of Osteopathic Medicine in Pennsylvania. Dr Rutt completed her Otolaryngology-Head and Neck Surgery Residency at the Detroit Medical Center in affiliation with Michigan State University. She

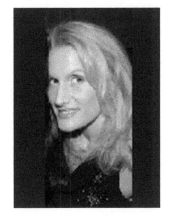

then completed an internationally renowned fellowship in laryngology and care of the professional voice at the prestigious American Institute for Voice and Ear Research in Philadelphia, in affiliation with Drexel University College of Medicine. Dr Rutt will be practicing Laryngology at the Mayo Clinic in Jacksonville, Florida.